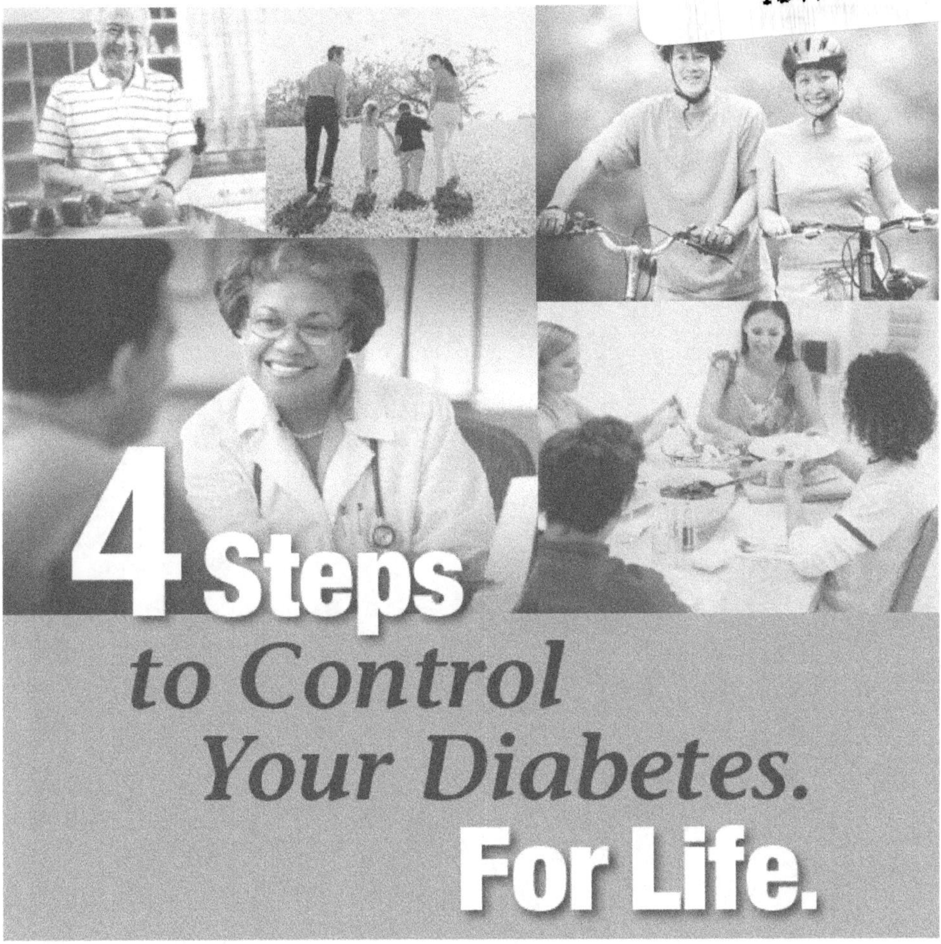

4 Steps

to Control
Your Diabetes.
For Life.

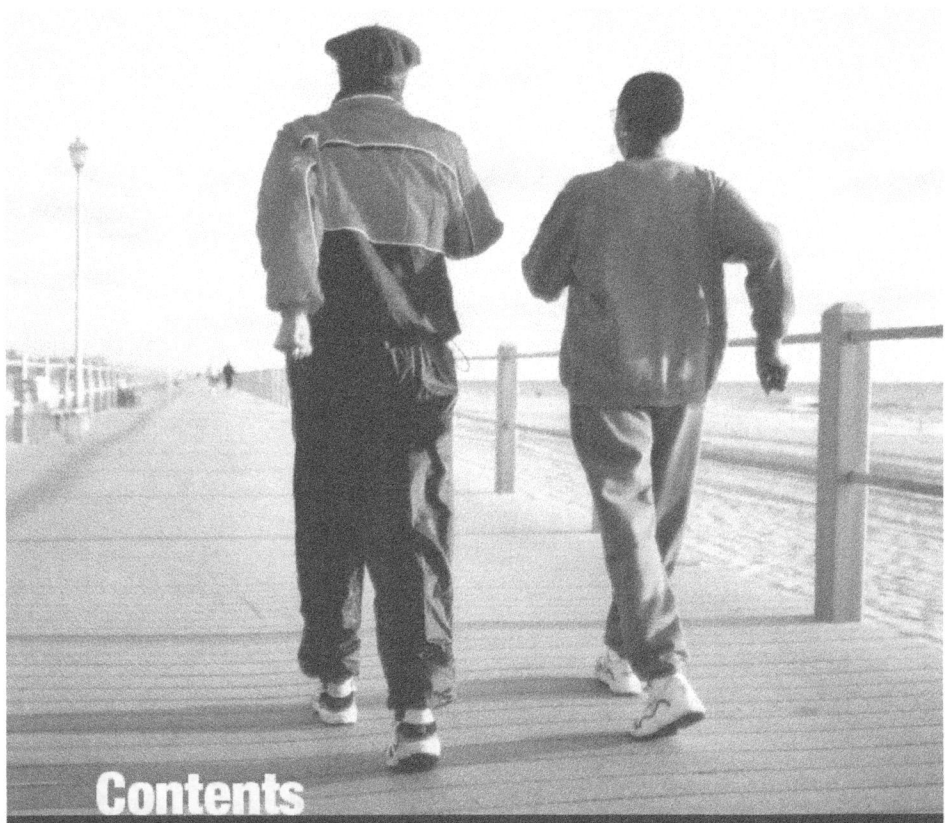

Contents

4 Steps to Control Your Diabetes. For Life.

This booklet presents four key steps to help you manage your diabetes and live a long and active life.

Step 1: Learn about diabetes.

Step 2: Know your diabetes ABCs.

Step 3: Manage your diabetes.

Step 4: Get routine care to avoid problems.

Diabetes is a serious disease. It affects almost every part of your body. That is why a health care team may help you take care of your diabetes:

- doctor
- diabetes educator
- eye doctor
- mental health counselor
- nurse practitioner
- social worker

- dentist
- dietitian
- foot doctor
- nurse
- pharmacist
- friends and family

You are the most important member of the team.

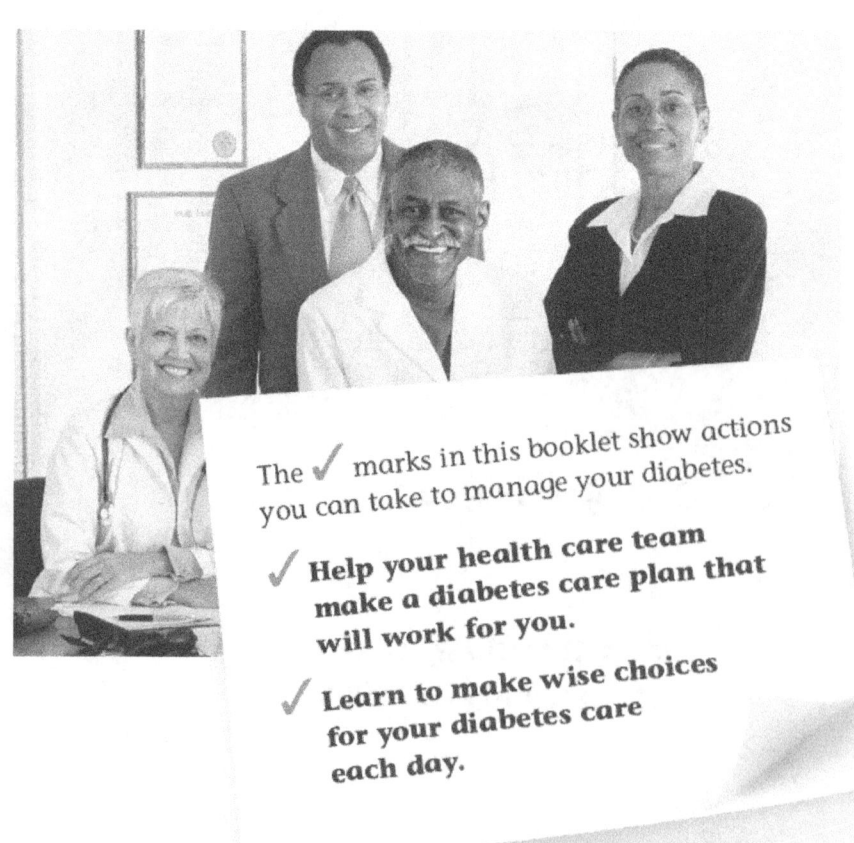

The ✓ marks in this booklet show actions you can take to manage your diabetes.

✓ Help your health care team make a diabetes care plan that will work for you.

✓ Learn to make wise choices for your diabetes care each day.

Step 1:
Learn about diabetes.

Diabetes means that your blood glucose (blood sugar) is too high. These are the main types of diabetes.

Type 1 diabetes — the body does not make insulin. Insulin helps the body use glucose from food for energy. People with type 1 need to take insulin every day.

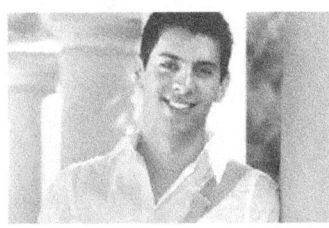

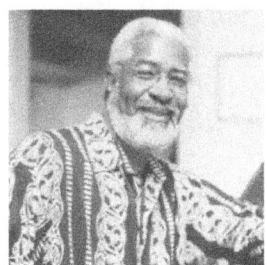

Type 2 diabetes — the body does not make or use insulin well. People with type 2 often need to take pills or insulin. Type 2 is the most common form of diabetes.

Gestational (jes-TAY-shon-al) diabetes — occurs in some women when they become pregnant. It raises her future risk of developing diabetes, mostly type 2. It may raise her child's risk of being overweight and developing type 2 diabetes.

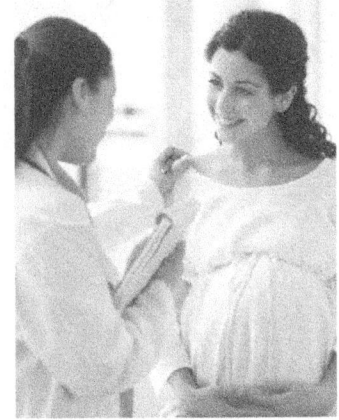

Diabetes is serious.

You may have heard people say they have "a touch of diabetes" or that their "sugar is a little high." These words suggest that diabetes is not a serious disease. That is **not** correct. Diabetes is serious, but you can learn to manage it!

It's Not Easy, But It's Worth It.

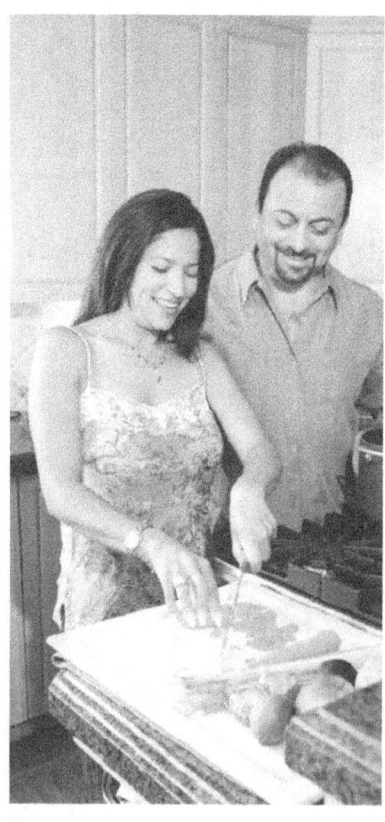

All people with diabetes need to make healthy food choices, stay at a healthy weight, and move more every day.

Taking good care of yourself and your diabetes can help you feel better. It may help you avoid health problems caused by diabetes such as:

- heart attack and stroke
- eye problems that can lead to trouble seeing or going blind
- nerve damage that can cause your hands and feet to hurt, tingle, or feel numb. Some people may even lose a foot or a leg
- kidney problems that can cause your kidneys to stop working
- gum disease and loss of teeth

4

When your blood glucose is close to normal you are likely to:

- have more energy
- be less tired and thirsty and urinate less often
- heal better and have fewer skin or bladder infections
- have fewer problems with your eyesight, feet, and gums

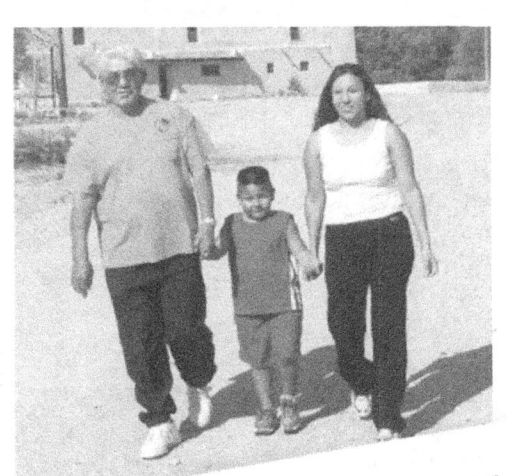

✓ Ask your health care team which type of diabetes you have.

✓ Learn why diabetes is serious.

✓ Learn how caring for your diabetes helps you feel better today and in the future.

Step 2:
Know your diabetes ABCs.

Talk to your health care team about how to manage your **A**1C, **B**lood pressure, and **C**holesterol. This can help lower your chances of having a heart attack, stroke, or other diabetes problems. Here's what the **ABCs** of diabetes stand for:

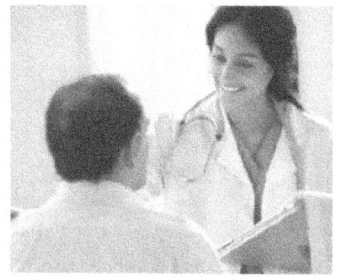

A for the A1C test (A-one-C).
It shows what your blood glucose has been over the last three months. The A1C goal for many people is below 7.

High blood glucose can harm your heart and blood vessels, kidneys, feet, and eyes.

B for Blood pressure.
The goal for most people with diabetes is below 130/80.

High blood pressure makes your heart work too hard. It can cause heart attack, stroke, and kidney disease.

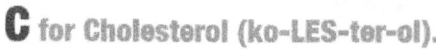

C for Cholesterol (ko-LES-ter-ol).
The LDL goal for people with diabetes is below 100.
The HDL for men is greater than 40.
The HDL for women is greater than 50.

LDL or "bad" cholesterol can build up and clog your blood vessels. It can cause a heart attack or a stroke. HDL or "good" cholesterol helps remove cholesterol from your blood vessels.

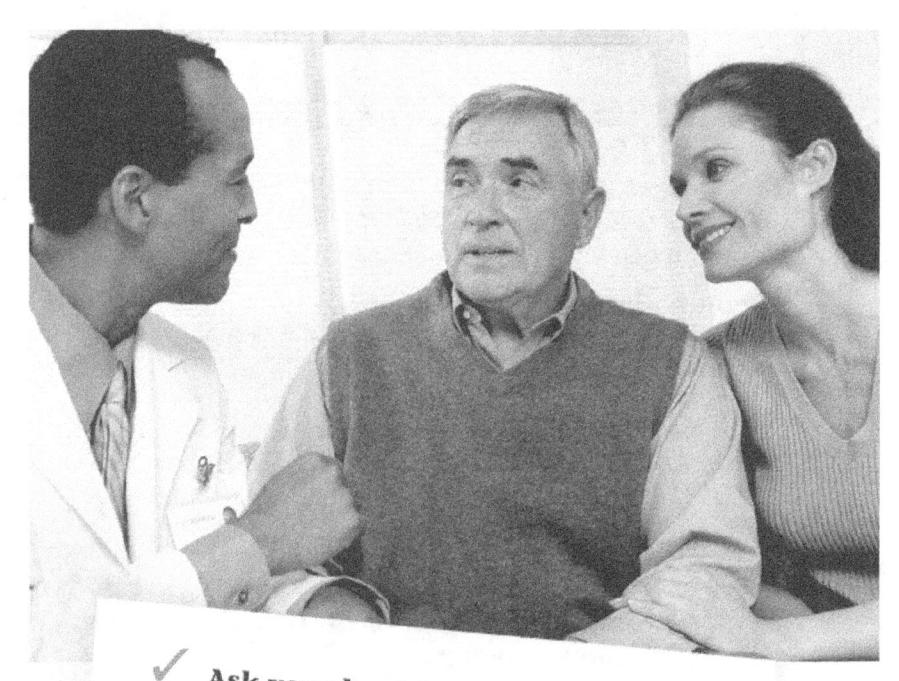

✓ **Ask your health care team:**

- what your A1C, blood pressure, and cholesterol numbers are
- what your A1C*, blood pressure, and cholesterol numbers <u>should be</u>
- what you can do to reach your targets

✓ **Write down all your numbers on the record card at the back of this booklet.**

* An A1C of less than 7 is the goal for many people but not for everyone. Talk to your health care team about what A1C target is right for you.

Step 3:
Manage your diabetes.

Many people avoid the long-term problems of diabetes by taking good care of themselves. Work with your health care team to reach your ABC target. Use this **self-care plan.**

- **Follow your diabetes meal plan.** If you do not have one, ask your health care team to help you develop a meal plan.

  - **Eat healthy foods** such as fruits and vegetables, fish, lean meats, chicken or turkey without the skin, dry peas or beans, whole grains, and low-fat or skim milk and cheese.

  - **Keep fish and lean meat and poultry portions to about 3 ounces** (or the size of a deck of cards). Bake, broil, or grill it.

  - **Eat foods that have less fat and salt.**

  - **Eat foods with more fiber** such as whole-grain cereals, breads, crackers, rice, or pasta.

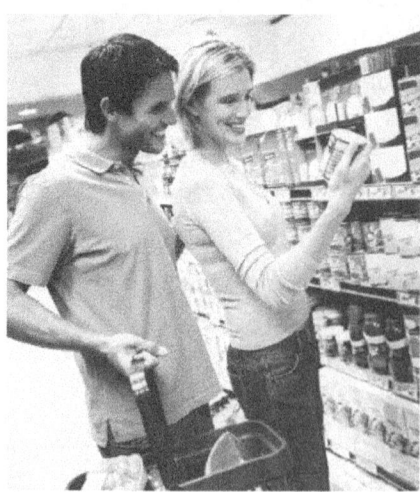

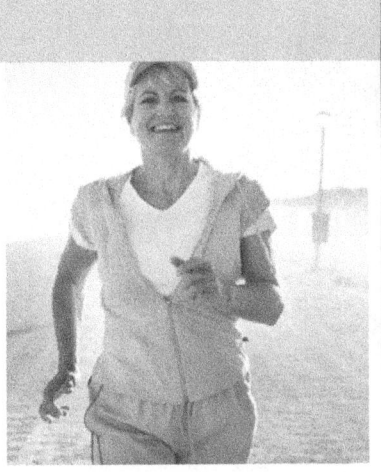
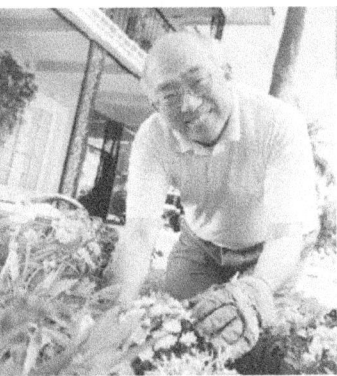

- **Get 30 to 60 minutes of physical activity** on most days of the week. Brisk walking is a great way to move more.

- **Stay at a healthy weight** by using your meal plan and moving more.

- **Ask for help if you feel down.** A mental health counselor, support group, member of the clergy, friend, or family member who will listen to your concerns may help you feel better.

- **Learn to cope with stress.** Stress can raise your blood glucose. While it is hard to remove stress from your life, you can learn to handle it. NDEP's Diabetes HealthSense provides online access to resources that support people with diabetes in making changes to live well. For more information visit www.YourDiabetesInfo.org/HealthSense.

- **Stop smoking.** Ask for help to quit. Call 1-800-QUITNOW(1-800-784-8669).

- **Take medicines even when you feel good.** Ask your doctor if you need **aspirin** to prevent a heart attack or stroke. Tell your doctor if you cannot afford your medicines or if you have any side effects.

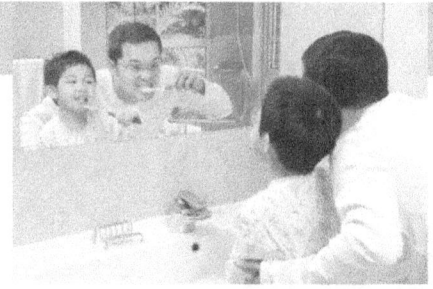

- **Check your feet every day** for cuts, blisters, red spots, and swelling. Call your health care team right away about any sores that do not go away.

- **Brush your teeth and floss every day** to avoid problems with your mouth, teeth, or gums.

- **Check your blood glucose.** You may want to test it one or more times a day. Use the card at the back of this booklet to keep a record of your blood glucose numbers. Be sure to show it to your health care team.

- **Check your blood pressure** if your doctor advises.

- **Report any changes in your eyesight** to your health care team.

✓ Talk to your health care team about your blood glucose targets. Ask how and when to test your blood glucose and how to use the results to manage your diabetes.

✓ Use this plan as a guide to your self-care.

✓ Discuss how your self-care plan is working for you each time you visit your health care team.

Step 4:
Get routine care.

See your health care team **at least twice a year** to find and treat any problems early.

At each visit be sure you have a:

- blood pressure check
- foot check
- weight check
- review of your self-care plan shown in Step 3

Two times each year have an:

- A1C test – it may be checked more often if it is over 7

Once each year be sure you have a:

- cholesterol test
- triglyceride (try-GLISS-er-ide) test — a type of blood fat
- complete foot exam
- dental exam to check teeth and gums — tell your dentist you have diabetes
- dilated eye exam to check for eye problems
- flu shot
- urine and a blood test to check for kidney problems

At least once get a:

- pneumonia (nu-mo-nya) shot

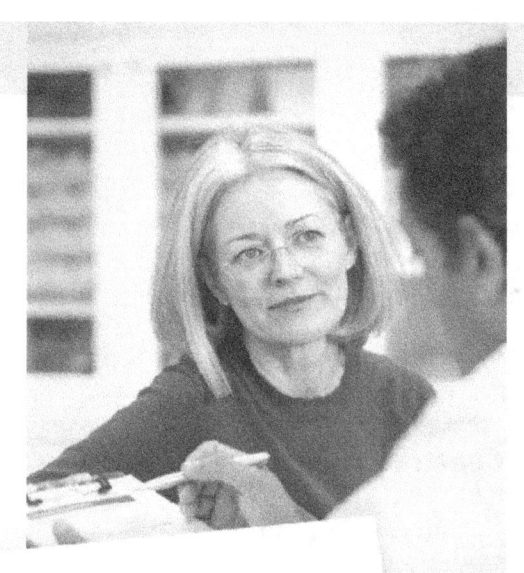

✓ Ask your health care team about these and other tests you may need. Ask what your results mean.

✓ Write down the date and time of your next visit.

✓ Use the card at the back of this booklet to keep a record of your diabetes care.

✓ If you have Medicare, ask your health care team if Medicare will cover some of the costs for

- learning about healthy eating and diabetes self-care
- special shoes, if you need them
- medical supplies
- diabetes medicines

My Diabetes Care Record

Record your targets and the date, time, and results of your tests. Take this card with you on your health care visits. Show it to your health care team to remind them of tests you need.

A1C — At least twice each year		Goal for many: below 7		My Target: _____	
Date					
Result					

Blood Pressure (BP) — Each visit		Goal for most: below 130/80		My Target: _____	
Date					
Result					

Cholesterol (LDL) — Once each year		Usual goal: below 100		My Target: _____	
Date					
Result					

Cholesterol (HDL) — Once each year		Usual goal: above 40		My Target: _____	
Date					
Result					

Triglycerides — Once each year		Usual goal: below 150		My Target: _____	
Date					
Result					

Weight — Each visit				My Target: _____	
Date					
Result					

TEAR HERE

NATIONAL DIABETES EDUCATION PROGRAM

www.YourDiabetesInfo.org

My Diabetes Care Record

	Date	Result
Each visit		
Foot check		
Review self-care plan		
Weight check		
Once a year		
Dental exam		
Dilated eye exam		
Complete foot exam		
Flu shot		
Kidney check		
At least once		
Pneumonia shot		

TEAR HERE

Self Checks of Blood Glucose

Record your targets and the date, time, and results of your checks. Take this card with you on your health care visits. Show it to your health care team.

Before meals: Usual goal 70 to 130 My Target: _____	1-2 hours after meals: Usual goal below 180 My Target: _____	Bedtime: Usual goal 110-150 My Target: _____

TEAR HERE

Notes:

_____
_____
_____
_____
_____
_____
_____
_____
_____
_____
_____
_____
_____
_____
_____
_____
_____
_____
_____

TEAR HERE

Where to get help:

Many of these groups offer items in English and Spanish.

American Association of Diabetes Educators
1-800-338-3633
www.diabeteseducator.org

American Diabetes Association
1-800-DIABETES (1-800-342-2383)
www.diabetes.org

American Dietetic Association
1-800-877-0877
www.eatright.org

American Heart Association
1-800-AHA-USA1 (1-800-242-8721)
www.americanheart.org

Centers for Disease Control and Prevention
1-800-CDC-INFO (1-800-232-4636)
www.cdc.gov/diabetes

Centers for Medicare & Medicaid Services
1-800-MEDICARE (1-800-633-4227)
www.medicare.gov/health/diabetes.asp

National Diabetes Education Program
1-888-693-NDEP (1-888-693-6337)
www.YourDiabetesInfo.org

National Diabetes Education Program: Diabetes HealthSense
An online library of resources for living well.
www.YourDiabetesInfo.org/HealthSense

National Institute of Diabetes and Digestive and Kidney Diseases
National Diabetes Information Clearinghouse
1-800-860-8747
www.niddk.nih.gov

National Kidney Disease Education Program
1-866-4-KIDNEY (1-866-454-3639)
www.nkdep.nih.gov

National Diabetes Education Program
1-888-693-NDEP (1-888-693-6337)
www.YourDiabetesInfo.org

The U.S. Department of Health and Human Services' National Diabetes Education Program (NDEP) is jointly sponsored by the **National Institutes of Health** (NIH) and the **Centers for Disease Control and Prevention** (CDC) with the support of more than 200 partner organizations.

Participants in research studies can play a more active role in improving their own health and help others by contributing to health-related research. See www.clinicaltrials.gov and www. cdc.gov/diabetes/projects/index.htm.

The NIDDK prints on recycled paper with bio-based ink.

Reviewed by Martha M. Funnell, MS, RN, CDE
Michigan Diabetes Research and Training Center

NIH Publication No. 11-5492 • May 2011

www.ingramcontent.com/pod-product-compliance
Lightning Source LLC
Chambersburg PA
CBHW071605170526
45166CB00004B/1807